Natural Medicine
First Aid Kit

Top Uses & Benefits

Natural Medicine
First Aid Kit

Recipe name:

Total Batch Volume:

Ingredient	Amount		Grams	Milliliters	Ounces	Pounds
		%				
		%				
		%				
		%				
		%				
		%				
		%				
		%				
		%				
		%				
		%				
		%				
		%				
Total	**100**	%				

Natural Medicine

First Aid Kit

Instructions

Natural Medicine

First Aid Kit

Notes

Natural Medicine
First Aid Kit

Top Uses & Benefits

Natural Medicine
First Aid Kit

Recipe name:

Total Batch Volume:

Ingredient	Amount		Grams	Milliliters	Ounces	Pounds
		%				
		%				
		%				
		%				
		%				
		%				
		%				
		%				
		%				
		%				
		%				
		%				
		%				
Total	100	%				

Natural Medicine

First Aid Kit

Instructions

Natural Medicine

First Aid Kit

Notes

Natural Medicine

First Aid Kit

Top Uses & Benefits

Natural Medicine
First Aid Kit

Recipe name:

Total Batch Volume:

Ingredient	Amount		Grams	Milliliters	Ounces	Pounds
		%				
		%				
		%				
		%				
		%				
		%				
		%				
		%				
		%				
		%				
		%				
		%				
		%				
Total	**100**	%				

Natural Medicine

First Aid Kit

Instructions

Natural Medicine
First Aid Kit

Notes

Natural Medicine
First Aid Kit

Top Uses & Benefits

Natural Medicine

First Aid Kit

Recipe name:

Total Batch Volume:

Ingredient	Amount		Grams	Milliliters	Ounces	Pounds
		%				
		%				
		%				
		%				
		%				
		%				
		%				
		%				
		%				
		%				
		%				
		%				
		%				
Total	**100**	%				

Natural Medicine
First Aid Kit

Instructions

Natural Medicine

First Aid Kit

Notes

Natural Medicine

First Aid Kit

Top Uses & Benefits

Natural Medicine
First Aid Kit

Recipe name:

Total Batch Volume:

Ingredient	Amount		Grams	Milliliters	Ounces	Pounds
		%				
		%				
		%				
		%				
		%				
		%				
		%				
		%				
		%				
		%				
		%				
		%				
		%				
Total	**100**	%				

Natural Medicine

First Aid Kit

Instructions

Natural Medicine

First Aid Kit

Notes

Natural Medicine

First Aid Kit

Top Uses & Benefits

Natural Medicine
First Aid Kit

Recipe name:

Total Batch Volume:

Ingredient	Amount		Grams	Milliliters	Ounces	Pounds
		%				
		%				
		%				
		%				
		%				
		%				
		%				
		%				
		%				
		%				
		%				
		%				
		%				
Total	**100**	%				

Natural Medicine

First Aid Kit

Instructions

Natural Medicine

First Aid Kit

Notes

Natural Medicine

First Aid Kit

Top Uses & Benefits

Natural Medicine
First Aid Kit

Recipe name:

Total Batch Volume:

Ingredient	Amount		Grams	Milliliters	Ounces	Pounds
		%				
		%				
		%				
		%				
		%				
		%				
		%				
		%				
		%				
		%				
		%				
		%				
		%				
Total	**100**	%				

Natural Medicine

First Aid Kit

Instructions

Natural Medicine

First Aid Kit

Notes

Natural Medicine

First Aid Kit

Top Uses & Benefits

Natural Medicine
First Aid Kit

Recipe name:

Total Batch Volume:

Ingredient	Amount		Grams	Milliliters	Ounces	Pounds
		%				
		%				
		%				
		%				
		%				
		%				
		%				
		%				
		%				
		%				
		%				
		%				
		%				
Total	**100**	%				

Natural Medicine

First Aid Kit

Instructions

Natural Medicine

First Aid Kit

Notes

Natural Medicine

First Aid Kit

Top Uses & Benefits

Natural Medicine
First Aid Kit

Recipe name:

Total Batch Volume:

Ingredient	Amount		Grams	Milliliters	Ounces	Pounds
		%				
		%				
		%				
		%				
		%				
		%				
		%				
		%				
		%				
		%				
		%				
		%				
		%				
Total	**100**	%				

Natural Medicine

First Aid Kit

Instructions

Natural Medicine

First Aid Kit

Notes

Natural Medicine
First Aid Kit

Top Uses & Benefits

Natural Medicine
First Aid Kit

Recipe name:

Total Batch Volume:

Ingredient	Amount		Grams	Milliliters	Ounces	Pounds
		%				
		%				
		%				
		%				
		%				
		%				
		%				
		%				
		%				
		%				
		%				
		%				
		%				
Total	**100**	%				

Natural Medicine
First Aid Kit

Instructions

Natural Medicine

First Aid Kit

Notes

Natural Medicine

First Aid Kit

Natural Medicine

First Aid Kit

www.ingramcontent.com/pod-product-compliance
Lightning Source LLC
Chambersburg PA
CBHW050846290526
45792CB00002B/538